My Kombucha Log

Right Track Publishing

Olathe, KS

My Kombucha Planner
Design and Writing © 2017 Tracy Tennant
Published by Right Track Publishing in 2017

righttrackpublishing.com

The information provided in this publication is for educational and record-keeping purposes only, and is not intended to replace professional medical or nutritional advice.

ISBN: 978-0-9913371-2-5

Kombucha Basics

Kombucha, or lightly fermented tea, is said to aid in digestion, promote gut bacteria, and support the immune system. Many legends exist about where and when Kombucha originated. We might never know how it began, but Kombucha has been around for at least a couple thousand years.

Buying pre-bottled Kombucha can get pretty expensive if you plan on drinking the beverage regularly. Making your own is a fun, simple, and cost-effective alternative.

You will need:

- ✔ A gallon-size glass container
- ✔ Cloth or coffee filters for cover
- ✔ Pot or kettle to boil water
- ✔ Spoon
- ✔ Funnel
- ✔ Strainer

For best results, it's recommended you follow the detailed directions from your favorite Kombucha book or website. Always take proper precautions for sanitary food preparation before brewing your Kombucha.

Ingredients:

6 - 8 bags organic black tea

1 cup sugar

1 gallon filtered water (minus 2 cups)

1 SCOBY

1 pint starter liquid (finished Kombucha)

It's best for beginners to stick with black tea. As you become more proficient at making Kombucha, you can experiment with different types of tea or blends of black, green, oolong, and white tea leaves. These types, along with pu-erh, all come from the Camellia sinensis plant. The main difference is in how the leaves are processed. Each type has its own unique health properties.

A SCOBY is a symbiotic culture of bacteria and yeast. Be sure to get a healthy SCOBY from a trusted source, such as a local Kombucha brewer (look online for your city). A healthy "mother" SCOBY should be 1/4 to 1/2-inch thick, and tan in color.

Heat two quarts of water to about 205 degrees, just below the boiling point. Add tea bags and let steep for 10 minutes. Remove tea bags. Add sugar and stir until dissolved. Cool to room temperature or maximum of 80 degrees. Transfer tea into your gallon glass jar along with enough remaining purified water to leave room for the SCOBY and starter liquid.

Using clean hands, gently pour the SCOBY and starter liquid into the jar, leaving about an inch of space at the top.

Cover with a coffee filter or clean cotton cloth (T-shirt material) and secure with a rubber band. Don't use cheesecloth; it's too porous and you don't want fruit flies to get in! Set the jar out of direct sunlight on your counter where it won't be disturbed or moved.

In three or four days you will notice a thin layer of new culture beginning to form on top. As the tea goes through its fermentation process, the new culture (SCOBY) will thicken. Fermentation takes 7 to 21 days depending on temperature and desired taste. The longer it sits, the more "bite" it will have. The ideal temperature for fermentation is 74 to 80 degrees. Anything below 73 degrees will take longer to ferment, resulting in slow SCOBY growth.

There isn't "one right way" or only one recipe to follow when home-brewing kombucha. Ingredients, proportions, and methods will vary. Experiment to find what works best for you. The important thing is to use clean hands and equipment, and to make sure your SCOBY is healthy. Anything that looks green, blue, red, black, or fuzzy is a sign of a bad batch. Throw it away and start over.

Flavorings should be added after the initial brew is finished. Herbs, spices, and a variety of fruit can be added to flavor the booch. Add pieces of good-quality fruit or spices to a clean, empty glass bottle (for example, diced organic fresh or frozen cherries, ginger, blueberries, etc.). Pour the newly finished kombucha into the bottle, almost to the top. Cap the bottle and let it sit at room temperature for one to three days. Be cautious opening the bottle in case carbonation has built up. Strain the kombucha, rebottle, refrigerate, and enjoy!

The resources below are great go-to's for beginners:

Websites

kombuchakamp.com

liveeatlearn.com/the-simple-guide-to-kickass-kombucha

Books

The Big Book of Kombucha: Brewing, Flavoring, and Enjoying the Health Benefits of Fermented Tea
by Hannah Crum and Alex LaGory

DIY Kombucha:
60 Nourishing Tonics for Health & Happiness
by Katherine Green

Keeping Track

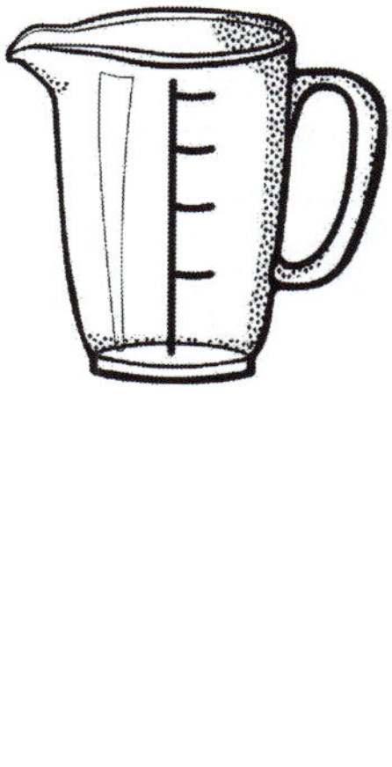

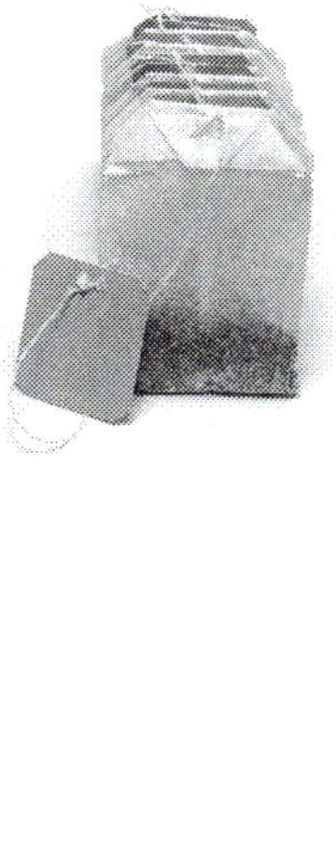

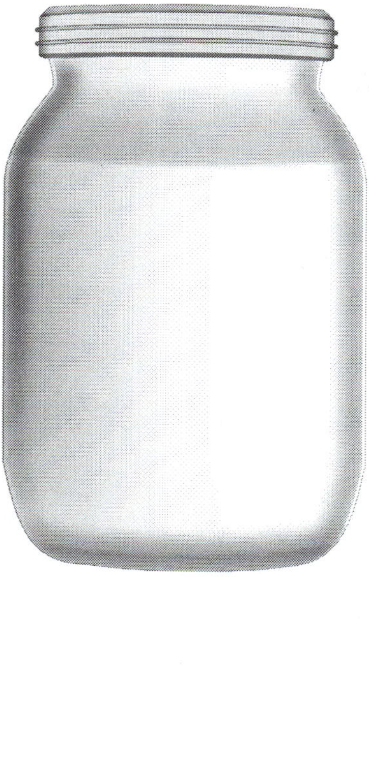

Details

Method: ☐ Batch ☐ Continuous

Vessel Size ________ Room Temp ______

Brew Date ______________________________

Tea Type ______________________________

Sugar Type ______________________________

☐ Day #____ Flavor____________________

☐ Day #____ Flavor____________________

☐ Day #____ Flavor____________________

☐ Day #____ Flavor____________________

Harvest Date ________________

Flavorings Added ________________________

____

Days for Second Ferment 1 2 3

Notes:

Details

Method: ☐ Batch ☐ Continuous

Vessel Size ________ Room Temp ______

Brew Date ______________________________

Tea Type ______________________________

Sugar Type ______________________________

☐ Day #_____ Flavor______________________

☐ Day #_____ Flavor______________________

☐ Day #_____ Flavor______________________

☐ Day #_____ Flavor______________________

Harvest Date ________________

Flavorings Added __________________________

____

Days for Second Ferment 1 2 3

Notes:

Details

Method: ☐ Batch ☐ Continuous

Vessel Size ________ Room Temp ______

Brew Date ______________________________

Tea Type ______________________________

Sugar Type ______________________________

☐ Day #_____ Flavor______________________

☐ Day #_____ Flavor______________________

☐ Day #_____ Flavor______________________

☐ Day #_____ Flavor______________________

Harvest Date ________________

Flavorings Added ________________________

____

Days for Second Ferment 1 2 3

Notes:

Details

Method: ☐ Batch ☐ Continuous

Vessel Size ________ Room Temp ______

Brew Date ______________________________

Tea Type ______________________________

Sugar Type ______________________________

☐ Day #____ Flavor____________________

☐ Day #____ Flavor____________________

☐ Day #____ Flavor____________________

☐ Day #____ Flavor____________________

Harvest Date ________________

Flavorings Added ________________________

____

Days for Second Ferment 1 2 3

Notes:

Details

Method: ☐ Batch ☐ Continuous

Vessel Size ________ Room Temp ______

Brew Date ______________________________

Tea Type ______________________________

Sugar Type ______________________________

☐ Day #____ Flavor____________________

☐ Day #____ Flavor____________________

☐ Day #____ Flavor____________________

☐ Day #____ Flavor____________________

Harvest Date ________________

Flavorings Added _________________________

____

Days for Second Ferment 1 2 3

Notes:

Details

Method: ☐ Batch ☐ Continuous

Vessel Size ________ Room Temp ______

Brew Date ______________________________

Tea Type ______________________________

Sugar Type ______________________________

☐ Day #_____ Flavor______________________

☐ Day #_____ Flavor______________________

☐ Day #_____ Flavor______________________

☐ Day #_____ Flavor______________________

Harvest Date ________________

Flavorings Added __________________________

____

Days for Second Ferment 1 2 3

Notes:

Details

Method: ☐ Batch ☐ Continuous

Vessel Size ________ Room Temp ______

Brew Date

Tea Type

Sugar Type

☐ Day #_____ Flavor______________________

☐ Day #_____ Flavor______________________

☐ Day #_____ Flavor______________________

☐ Day #_____ Flavor______________________

Harvest Date

Flavorings Added ___________________________

____

Days for Second Ferment 1 2 3

Notes:

Details

Method: ☐ Batch ☐ Continuous

Vessel Size ________ Room Temp ______

Brew Date ______________________________

Tea Type ______________________________

Sugar Type ______________________________

☐ Day #_____ Flavor_____________________

☐ Day #_____ Flavor_____________________

☐ Day #_____ Flavor_____________________

☐ Day #_____ Flavor_____________________

Harvest Date ________________

Flavorings Added __________________________

____

Days for Second Ferment 1 2 3

Notes:

Details

Method: ☐ Batch ☐ Continuous

Vessel Size ________ Room Temp ______

Brew Date ______________________________

Tea Type ______________________________

Sugar Type ______________________________

☐ Day #_____ Flavor______________________

☐ Day #_____ Flavor______________________

☐ Day #_____ Flavor______________________

☐ Day #_____ Flavor______________________

Harvest Date ________________

Flavorings Added __________________________

____

Days for Second Ferment 1 2 3

Notes:

Details

Method: ☐ Batch ☐ Continuous

Vessel Size ________ Room Temp ______

Brew Date

Tea Type

Sugar Type

☐ Day #_____ Flavor______________________

☐ Day #_____ Flavor______________________

☐ Day #_____ Flavor______________________

☐ Day #_____ Flavor______________________

Harvest Date

Flavorings Added ___________________________

____

Days for Second Ferment 1 2 3

Notes:

Details

Method: ☐ Batch ☐ Continuous

Vessel Size ________ Room Temp ______

Brew Date ________________________________

Tea Type ________________________________

Sugar Type ________________________________

☐ Day #_____ Flavor______________________

☐ Day #_____ Flavor______________________

☐ Day #_____ Flavor______________________

☐ Day #_____ Flavor______________________

Harvest Date ________________

Flavorings Added __________________________

____

Days for Second Ferment 1 2 3

Notes:

Details

Method: ☐ Batch ☐ Continuous

Vessel Size _______ Room Temp _____

Brew Date ____________________

Tea Type ____________________

Sugar Type ____________________

☐ Day #____ Flavor__________________

☐ Day #____ Flavor__________________

☐ Day #____ Flavor__________________

☐ Day #____ Flavor__________________

Harvest Date ____________

Flavorings Added ______________________

____

Days for Second Ferment 1 2 3

Notes:

Details

Method: ☐ Batch ☐ Continuous

Vessel Size ________ Room Temp ______

Brew Date ______________________________

Tea Type ______________________________

Sugar Type ______________________________

☐ Day #____ Flavor____________________

☐ Day #____ Flavor____________________

☐ Day #____ Flavor____________________

☐ Day #____ Flavor____________________

Harvest Date ________________

Flavorings Added _________________________

____

Days for Second Ferment 1 2 3

Notes:

Details

Method: ☐ Batch ☐ Continuous

Vessel Size _______ Room Temp _____

Brew Date

Tea Type

Sugar Type

☐ Day #____ Flavor__________________

☐ Day #____ Flavor__________________

☐ Day #____ Flavor__________________

☐ Day #____ Flavor__________________

Harvest Date

Flavorings Added ______________________

____

Days for Second Ferment 1 2 3

Notes:

Details

Method: ☐ Batch ☐ Continuous

Vessel Size ________ Room Temp ______

Brew Date ________________

Tea Type ________________

Sugar Type ________________

☐ Day #____ Flavor ______________________

☐ Day #____ Flavor ______________________

☐ Day #____ Flavor ______________________

☐ Day #____ Flavor ______________________

Harvest Date ____________

Flavorings Added ____________________________

____

Days for Second Ferment 1 2 3

Notes:

Details

Method: ☐ Batch ☐ Continuous

Vessel Size ________ Room Temp ______

Brew Date ________________________________

Tea Type ________________________________

Sugar Type ________________________________

☐ Day #_____ Flavor______________________

☐ Day #_____ Flavor______________________

☐ Day #_____ Flavor______________________

☐ Day #_____ Flavor______________________

Harvest Date ________________

Flavorings Added ___________________________

____

Days for Second Ferment 1 2 3

Notes:

Details

Method: ☐ Batch ☐ Continuous

Vessel Size ________ Room Temp ______

Brew Date

Tea Type

Sugar Type

☐ Day #_____ Flavor_____________________

☐ Day #_____ Flavor_____________________

☐ Day #_____ Flavor_____________________

☐ Day #_____ Flavor_____________________

Harvest Date

Flavorings Added _________________________

____

Days for Second Ferment 1 2 3

Notes:

Details

Method: ☐ Batch ☐ Continuous

Vessel Size ________ Room Temp ______

Brew Date ______________________________

Tea Type ______________________________

Sugar Type ______________________________

☐ Day #_____ Flavor______________________

☐ Day #_____ Flavor______________________

☐ Day #_____ Flavor______________________

☐ Day #_____ Flavor______________________

Harvest Date ________________

Flavorings Added _________________________

____

Days for Second Ferment 1 2 3

Notes:

Details

Method: ☐ Batch ☐ Continuous

Vessel Size ________ Room Temp ______

Brew Date

Tea Type

Sugar Type

☐ Day #_____ Flavor______________________

☐ Day #_____ Flavor______________________

☐ Day #_____ Flavor______________________

☐ Day #_____ Flavor______________________

Harvest Date

Flavorings Added __________________________

____

Days for Second Ferment 1 2 3

Notes:

Details

Method: ☐ Batch ☐ Continuous

Vessel Size ________ Room Temp _____

Brew Date

Tea Type

Sugar Type

☐ Day #____ Flavor____________________

☐ Day #____ Flavor____________________

☐ Day #____ Flavor____________________

☐ Day #____ Flavor____________________

Harvest Date

Flavorings Added ________________________

____

Days for Second Ferment 1 2 3

Notes:

Details

Method: ☐ Batch ☐ Continuous

Vessel Size ________ Room Temp ______

Brew Date

Tea Type

Sugar Type

☐ Day #____ Flavor____________________

☐ Day #____ Flavor____________________

☐ Day #____ Flavor____________________

☐ Day #____ Flavor____________________

Harvest Date

Flavorings Added ________________________

____

Days for Second Ferment 1 2 3

Notes:

Details

Method: ☐ Batch ☐ Continuous

Vessel Size _______ Room Temp _____

Brew Date

Tea Type

Sugar Type

☐ Day #____ Flavor__________________

☐ Day #____ Flavor__________________

☐ Day #____ Flavor__________________

☐ Day #____ Flavor__________________

Harvest Date

Flavorings Added ______________________

____

Days for Second Ferment 1 2 3

Notes:

Details

Method: ☐ Batch ☐ Continuous

Vessel Size ________ Room Temp ______

Brew Date

Tea Type

Sugar Type

☐ Day #_____ Flavor______________________

☐ Day #_____ Flavor______________________

☐ Day #_____ Flavor______________________

☐ Day #_____ Flavor______________________

Harvest Date

Flavorings Added ___________________________

____

Days for Second Ferment 1 2 3

Notes:

Details

Method: ☐ Batch ☐ Continuous

Vessel Size _______ Room Temp _____

Brew Date ____________________

Tea Type ____________________

Sugar Type ____________________

☐ Day #____ Flavor ____________________

☐ Day #____ Flavor ____________________

☐ Day #____ Flavor ____________________

☐ Day #____ Flavor ____________________

Harvest Date ____________

Flavorings Added ____________________

____

Days for Second Ferment 1 2 3

Notes:

Details

Method: ☐ Batch ☐ Continuous

Vessel Size ________ Room Temp ______

Brew Date

Tea Type

Sugar Type

☐ Day #____ Flavor____________________

☐ Day #____ Flavor____________________

☐ Day #____ Flavor____________________

☐ Day #____ Flavor____________________

Harvest Date

Flavorings Added ________________________

____

Days for Second Ferment 1 2 3

Notes:

Details

Method: ☐ Batch ☐ Continuous

Vessel Size ________ Room Temp ______

Brew Date ______________________________

Tea Type ______________________________

Sugar Type ______________________________

☐ Day #_____ Flavor______________________

☐ Day #_____ Flavor______________________

☐ Day #_____ Flavor______________________

☐ Day #_____ Flavor______________________

Harvest Date ________________

Flavorings Added __________________________

____

Days for Second Ferment 1 2 3

Notes:

Details

Method: ☐ Batch ☐ Continuous

Vessel Size ________ Room Temp ______

Brew Date

Tea Type

Sugar Type

☐ Day #_____ Flavor______________________

☐ Day #_____ Flavor______________________

☐ Day #_____ Flavor______________________

☐ Day #_____ Flavor______________________

Harvest Date

Flavorings Added ___________________________

____

Days for Second Ferment 1 2 3

Notes:

Details

Method: ☐ Batch ☐ Continuous

Vessel Size ________ Room Temp ______

Brew Date ______________________________

Tea Type ______________________________

Sugar Type ______________________________

☐ Day #_____ Flavor_____________________

☐ Day #_____ Flavor_____________________

☐ Day #_____ Flavor_____________________

☐ Day #_____ Flavor_____________________

Harvest Date ________________

Flavorings Added __________________________

____

Days for Second Ferment 1 2 3

Notes:

Details

Method: ☐ Batch ☐ Continuous

Vessel Size ________ Room Temp ______

Brew Date ________________________________

Tea Type ________________________________

Sugar Type ________________________________

☐ Day #_____ Flavor______________________

☐ Day #_____ Flavor______________________

☐ Day #_____ Flavor______________________

☐ Day #_____ Flavor______________________

Harvest Date ________________

Flavorings Added ___________________________

____

Days for Second Ferment 1 2 3

Notes:

Details

Method: ☐ Batch ☐ Continuous

Vessel Size _______ Room Temp _____

Brew Date

Tea Type

Sugar Type

☐ Day #____ Flavor__________________

☐ Day #____ Flavor__________________

☐ Day #____ Flavor__________________

☐ Day #____ Flavor__________________

Harvest Date

Flavorings Added ______________________

____

Days for Second Ferment 1 2 3

Notes:

Details

Method: ☐ Batch ☐ Continuous

Vessel Size _______ Room Temp _____

Brew Date ____________________

Tea Type ____________________

Sugar Type ____________________

☐ Day #____ Flavor__________________

☐ Day #____ Flavor__________________

☐ Day #____ Flavor__________________

☐ Day #____ Flavor__________________

Harvest Date ____________

Flavorings Added ______________________

____

Days for Second Ferment 1 2 3

Notes:

Details

Method: ☐ Batch ☐ Continuous

Vessel Size ________ Room Temp _____

Brew Date ______________________________

Tea Type ______________________________

Sugar Type ______________________________

☐ Day #____ Flavor____________________

☐ Day #____ Flavor____________________

☐ Day #____ Flavor____________________

☐ Day #____ Flavor____________________

Harvest Date ________________

Flavorings Added ________________________

____

Days for Second Ferment 1 2 3

Notes:

Details

Method: ☐ Batch ☐ Continuous

Vessel Size ________ Room Temp ______

Brew Date

Tea Type

Sugar Type

☐ Day #_____ Flavor______________________

☐ Day #_____ Flavor______________________

☐ Day #_____ Flavor______________________

☐ Day #_____ Flavor______________________

Harvest Date

Flavorings Added ___________________________

____

Days for Second Ferment 1 2 3

Notes:

Details

Method: ☐ Batch ☐ Continuous

Vessel Size ________ Room Temp _____

Brew Date ______________________________

Tea Type ______________________________

Sugar Type ______________________________

☐ Day #_____ Flavor______________________

☐ Day #_____ Flavor______________________

☐ Day #_____ Flavor______________________

☐ Day #_____ Flavor______________________

Harvest Date ________________

Flavorings Added __________________________

____

Days for Second Ferment 1 2 3

Notes:

Details

Method: ☐ Batch ☐ Continuous

Vessel Size ________ Room Temp ______

Brew Date ____________________

Tea Type ____________________

Sugar Type ____________________

☐ Day #_____ Flavor______________________

☐ Day #_____ Flavor______________________

☐ Day #_____ Flavor______________________

☐ Day #_____ Flavor______________________

Harvest Date ______________

Flavorings Added ___________________________

____

Days for Second Ferment 1 2 3

Notes:

Details

Method: ☐ Batch ☐ Continuous

Vessel Size ________ Room Temp _____

Brew Date ______________________________

Tea Type ______________________________

Sugar Type ______________________________

☐ Day #____ Flavor____________________

☐ Day #____ Flavor____________________

☐ Day #____ Flavor____________________

☐ Day #____ Flavor____________________

Harvest Date ________________

Flavorings Added ________________________

____

Days for Second Ferment 1 2 3

Notes:

Details

Method: ☐ Batch ☐ Continuous

Vessel Size ________ Room Temp ______

Brew Date ____________________

Tea Type ____________________

Sugar Type ____________________

☐ Day #____ Flavor____________________

☐ Day #____ Flavor____________________

☐ Day #____ Flavor____________________

☐ Day #____ Flavor____________________

Harvest Date ______________

Flavorings Added ____________________

____

Days for Second Ferment 1 2 3

Notes:

Details

Method: ☐ Batch ☐ Continuous

Vessel Size _______ Room Temp _____

Brew Date

Tea Type

Sugar Type

☐ Day #____ Flavor__________________

☐ Day #____ Flavor__________________

☐ Day #____ Flavor__________________

☐ Day #____ Flavor__________________

Harvest Date

Flavorings Added ______________________

____

Days for Second Ferment 1 2 3

Notes:

Details

Method: ☐ Batch ☐ Continuous

Vessel Size ________ Room Temp ______

Brew Date

Tea Type

Sugar Type

☐ Day #_____ Flavor______________________

☐ Day #_____ Flavor______________________

☐ Day #_____ Flavor______________________

☐ Day #_____ Flavor______________________

Harvest Date

Flavorings Added ___________________________

____

Days for Second Ferment 1 2 3

Notes:

Details

Method: ☐ Batch ☐ Continuous

Vessel Size ________ Room Temp ______

Brew Date ______________________________

Tea Type ______________________________

Sugar Type ______________________________

☐ Day #____ Flavor____________________

☐ Day #____ Flavor____________________

☐ Day #____ Flavor____________________

☐ Day #____ Flavor____________________

Harvest Date ________________

Flavorings Added _________________________

____

Days for Second Ferment 1 2 3

Notes:

Details

Method: ☐ Batch ☐ Continuous

Vessel Size ________ Room Temp ______

Brew Date ______________________________

Tea Type ______________________________

Sugar Type ______________________________

☐ Day #____ Flavor____________________

☐ Day #____ Flavor____________________

☐ Day #____ Flavor____________________

☐ Day #____ Flavor____________________

Harvest Date ________________

Flavorings Added ________________________

____

Days for Second Ferment 1 2 3

Notes:

Details

Method: ☐ Batch ☐ Continuous

Vessel Size _______ Room Temp _____

Brew Date

Tea Type

Sugar Type

☐ Day #____ Flavor__________________

☐ Day #____ Flavor__________________

☐ Day #____ Flavor__________________

☐ Day #____ Flavor__________________

Harvest Date

Flavorings Added ______________________

____

Days for Second Ferment 1 2 3

Notes:

Details

Method: ☐ Batch ☐ Continuous

Vessel Size ________ Room Temp ______

Brew Date

Tea Type

Sugar Type

☐ Day #_____ Flavor______________________

☐ Day #_____ Flavor______________________

☐ Day #_____ Flavor______________________

☐ Day #_____ Flavor______________________

Harvest Date

Flavorings Added ___________________________

____

Days for Second Ferment 1 2 3

Notes:

Details

Method: ☐ Batch ☐ Continuous

Vessel Size ________ Room Temp ______

Brew Date ______________________________

Tea Type ______________________________

Sugar Type ______________________________

☐ Day #____ Flavor____________________

☐ Day #____ Flavor____________________

☐ Day #____ Flavor____________________

☐ Day #____ Flavor____________________

Harvest Date ________________

Flavorings Added ________________________

____

Days for Second Ferment 1 2 3

Notes:

Details

Method: ☐ Batch ☐ Continuous

Vessel Size ________ Room Temp ______

Brew Date

Tea Type

Sugar Type

☐ Day #_____ Flavor______________________

☐ Day #_____ Flavor______________________

☐ Day #_____ Flavor______________________

☐ Day #_____ Flavor______________________

Harvest Date

Flavorings Added ___________________________

____

Days for Second Ferment 1 2 3

Notes:

Details

Method: ☐ Batch ☐ Continuous

Vessel Size _______ Room Temp _____

Brew Date

Tea Type

Sugar Type

☐ Day #____ Flavor__________________

☐ Day #____ Flavor__________________

☐ Day #____ Flavor__________________

☐ Day #____ Flavor__________________

Harvest Date

Flavorings Added ______________________

____

Days for Second Ferment 1 2 3

Notes:

Details

Method: ☐ Batch ☐ Continuous

Vessel Size ________ Room Temp ______

Brew Date

Tea Type

Sugar Type

☐ Day #_____ Flavor______________________

☐ Day #_____ Flavor______________________

☐ Day #_____ Flavor______________________

☐ Day #_____ Flavor______________________

Harvest Date

Flavorings Added ___________________________

____

Days for Second Ferment 1 2 3

Notes:

Details

Method: ☐ Batch ☐ Continuous

Vessel Size ________ Room Temp ______

Brew Date ________________________________

Tea Type ________________________________

Sugar Type ________________________________

☐ Day #_____ Flavor______________________

☐ Day #_____ Flavor______________________

☐ Day #_____ Flavor______________________

☐ Day #_____ Flavor______________________

Harvest Date __________________

Flavorings Added ___________________________

____

Days for Second Ferment 1 2 3

Notes:

Details

Method: ☐ Batch ☐ Continuous

Vessel Size ________ Room Temp ______

Brew Date ______________________________

Tea Type ______________________________

Sugar Type ______________________________

☐ Day #_____ Flavor______________________

☐ Day #_____ Flavor______________________

☐ Day #_____ Flavor______________________

☐ Day #_____ Flavor______________________

Harvest Date ________________

Flavorings Added ________________________

____

Days for Second Ferment 1 2 3

Notes:

Details

Method: ☐ Batch ☐ Continuous

Vessel Size ________ Room Temp ______

Brew Date ______________________________

Tea Type ______________________________

Sugar Type ______________________________

☐ Day #_____ Flavor______________________

☐ Day #_____ Flavor______________________

☐ Day #_____ Flavor______________________

☐ Day #_____ Flavor______________________

Harvest Date ________________

Flavorings Added __________________________

____

Days for Second Ferment 1 2 3

Notes: